BARBITURATES AND OTHER DEPRESSANTS

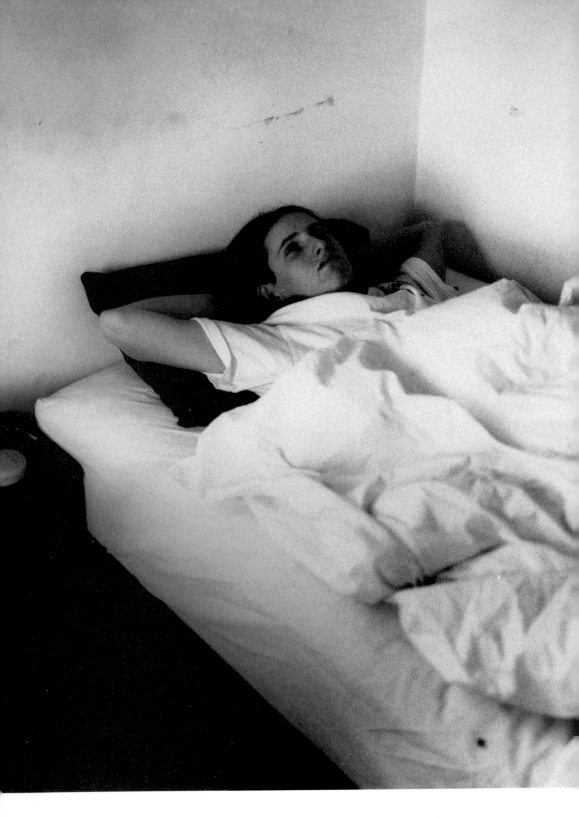

Depressants can change your personality and destroy your life.

BARBITURATES AND OTHER DEPRESSANTS

Lawrence Clayton, Ph.D.

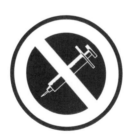

THE ROSEN PUBLISHING GROUP, INC.

NEW YORK

To Gary Cone

The people pictured in this book are only models; they in no way practice or endorse the activities illustrated. Captions serve only to explain the subjects of the photographs and do not imply a connection between real-life models and the staged situations shown. News agency photographs are exceptions.

Published in 1994, 1998 by The Rosen Publishing Group, Inc.
29 East 21st Street, New York, NY 10010

Copyright 1994, 1998 by The Rosen Publishing Group, Inc.

Revised Edition 1998

Library of Congress Cataloging-in-Publication Data

Clayton, L. (Lawrence)
   Barbiturates and other depressants / by Lawrence Clayton.
      p.   cm.—(The Drug abuse prevention library)
   Includes bibliographical references and index.
   ISBN 0-8239-2601-X
   1. Teenagers—Drug use—United States—Juvenile literature.   2. Drug abuse—United States—Juvenile literature.   3. Barbiturates—Juvenile literature.
   4. Central nervous system depressants—Juvenile literature.   [1. Drug abuse.   2. Barbiturates.
   3. Alcoholism.]   I. Title.   II. Series.
   HV5824.Y68C59   1994
   362.29′9—dc20   93-46270
                                                       CIP
                                                       AC

Manufactured in the United States of America

Contents

Introduction

Robert had always thought of Jeremy as his best friend. But lately, Jeremy was acting like a completely different person. Whenever they were together, Jeremy always brought along his "downers." At first he had taken them only at parties, but lately he was taking them every day. Jeremy always tried to persuade Robert to take some, too. Jeremy talked about how relaxed he felt when he took the pills.

Robert was shy and a bit of a loner. He started to think that maybe a few downers would help him be more outgoing. Maybe they would help him ask out this girl he liked. Jeremy never seemed to be nervous, even around the most popular girls in school.

But seeing Jeremy when he hadn't taken the downers for a while made Robert think it wasn't such a good idea after all. Jeremy could hardly sit still. He acted nervous and complained of feeling sick. Robert knew that Jeremy couldn't sleep without taking the pills, either. Lately, it seemed that he couldn't do anything without them. It was as if Jeremy couldn't live without them. He started cutting school. Sometimes, Robert would skip classes too because he couldn't say no to Jeremy. It was getting harder and harder to hang out with Jeremy and his friends and not be tempted to take drugs. Robert didn't know what to do. He didn't have any other friends to turn to for support, and he wasn't really confident enough to break from the group and risk losing his best friend.

Many teenagers today have to deal with a lot of pressure and stress. School, friends, and parents may pull you in different directions as you try to discover who you are. As you grow older, you learn to handle the stress of everyday life. Whether you feel frustrated, confused, angry, or hurt, it's important to face those feelings. By confronting your problems, you are better able to handle many of life's challenges. Unfortunately, like

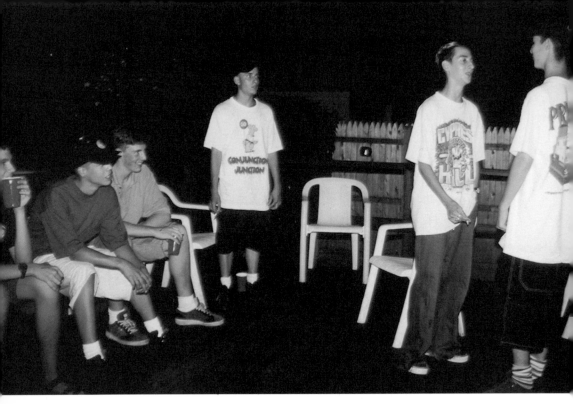

Teens may try a drug to fit in with a certain group of friends.

Jeremy, many teens turn to drugs and alcohol to try to make the problems go away. Drugs and alcohol, however, only make the problems worse.

This book is about depressants. Depressant drugs include barbiturates, benzodiazepines, and alcohol. Depressants can be very dangerous when they are abused. Abusers of these drugs can become addicted quickly. Stopping the abuse is difficult and often dangerous. It's important to understand the dangers involved in taking depressants. They cause thousands of deaths each year in the United States. People who understand the great risks are more likely to decide not to abuse them.

9

In this book we will talk about the different kinds of depressants. You will learn what these drugs are, their street names, where they come from, and what happens to your life and your body when you abuse them. Most important, this book will discuss how to get help if you or someone you care about becomes addicted.

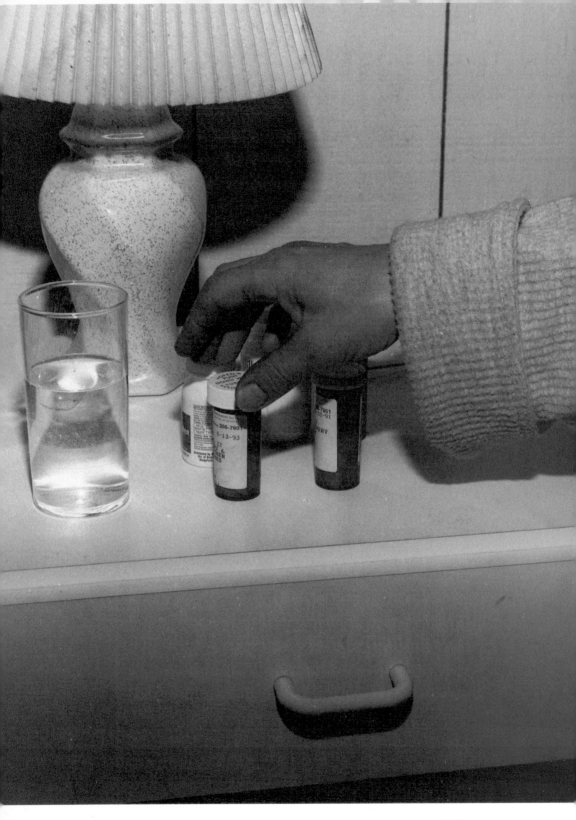

Many people rely on medication to help them relax and fall asleep.

CHAPTER 1

What Are Drug Abuse and Drug Addiction?

*T*here are different stages of drug abuse and addiction. Not everyone who takes drugs becomes an abuser or an addict. But many people cannot control their drug use. Some people are more likely to become addicted than others. It is important to know the risks before you start experimenting with drugs.

Who's at Risk?

Some research suggests that drug addiction is genetic. That is, you may be at a higher risk for drug abuse if your parents abuse drugs. Drug addiction is a disease. If someone in your family suffers from drug addiction, it does not automatically

11

12 | make you an addict. But your chances of developing an addiction are increased. It's something to be aware of before you take any drug.

Many teens learn how to cope with problems from watching their parents. You may have had your first encounter with drugs in the home by seeing your parent drink alcohol. Your parent may drink responsibly, and drinking itself may seem to you like a harmless way to cope with difficult situations.

Often, when a teen starts using a drug, he or she doesn't think it will become a problem. You may believe that you can handle it. Your friends may pressure you into trying drugs. You may think that drugs won't hurt you, but taking drugs is dangerous and can lead to abuse and addiction.

Teens usually start taking drugs at a party or when hanging out with friends. You may try a drug because someone tells you it will make you feel good. You may try a drink or take a pill because you feel uncomfortable or nervous and need to relax. You may think it's safe because everyone else is doing it. But taking drugs is not safe. Using any drug, even once, can be dangerous.

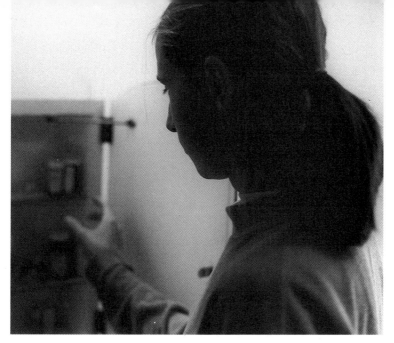

Parents may be unaware that their own pills pose a threat to an unstable teenage son or daughter.

Tolerance

If you continue taking drugs, your body soon develops a tolerance for them. Tolerance means that you need to use more and more of the drug to get the original effect. For example, at first, a couple of drinks may be all you need to feel good. But soon you find that you need much more than that to get the same feeling.

The longer you use a drug, the more you need to increase the amount you take.

Abuse

What began as casual use at parties with friends becomes a common occurrence. Soon, the drug use progresses and

13

14 becomes a habit. Drugs are always around and a part of every activity. When people arrange their lives and activities around their drug use, they have crossed the line from use to abuse. Drugs become more and more important. At this stage, drugs start to cause major trouble in the user's life.

Addiction

The longer a person abuses a drug, the greater the chance that he or she will become addicted. Addiction means completely losing control over how much you use or how often you use. When a person is addicted to drugs, he or she cannot stop using. An addict will steal and lie and hurt people to get drugs.

Addiction results from psychological and physical dependence. Psychological dependence means that a person *thinks* he or she needs the drug in order to function.

Physical dependence means that a person's *body* needs the drug to function and experiences withdrawal symptoms without it. These symptoms include nausea, sweating, confusion, depression, insomnia, chills, cramps, and disorientation.

An addict cares only about getting drugs and maintaining the supply. The drug becomes the most important thing in an addict's life. An addict cannot stop using on his or her own and needs professional help to quit.

Later, we will discuss what kind of medical treatment is necessary to quit successfully. One thing is clear: Drug abuse and drug addiction can ruin your life. By choosing not to use drugs, you are choosing to enjoy life and all it can offer.

15

CHAPTER 2

Teens and Drug Abuse

*O*ne weekend, Rachel was at the home of
her boyfriend, Eric. He had invited a few
friends to come over while his parents were
away. When the friends arrived, Rachel could
tell that all of them had been drinking. They
also had brought some beer with them to
Eric's house. Soon Rachel and Eric were
drinking too.

That night, after Rachel had had several
beers, she saw Eric's friend Paul passing
around some pills he called "red devils." Eric
had already taken a few and was sitting
silently on the floor, looking like he was only
half awake. Paul offered some "red devils"
to Rachel. Even though Rachel wasn't sure
what they were or what they would do, she
swallowed the pills.

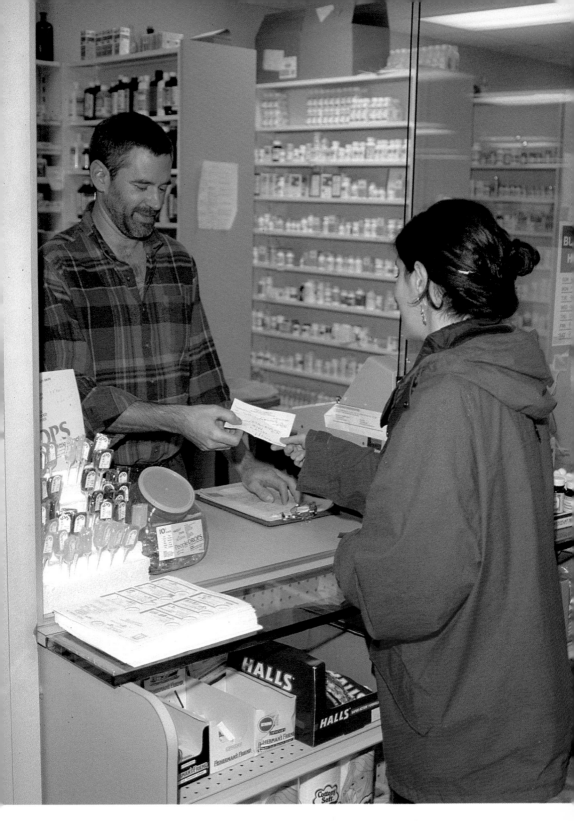

Your pharmacist will be happy to answer questions about medication prescribed for you by your doctor.

18 | *The next day at school, Rachel saw her friend Carla, who had also been at Eric's party. "How are you feeling?" Carla asked. "When I left Eric's house, you looked a little sick."*

"Well, I really felt awful this morning," Rachel replied. "But what's worse is what happened later last night. By the time everyone else had gone, Eric and I weren't thinking very clearly. We had sex, but we were so careless that we forgot to use protection. Now I'm really scared. I don't know what I'll do if I'm pregnant."

Teen drug abuse is a growing problem. Teenagers are encountering drugs at younger ages than ever before. It is difficult to cope with all the changes that are happening in your body and in your life. Making the right decision about drugs or sex is not always easy. But knowing what is right for you and how to say no if something makes you uncomfortable is an important skill everyone needs to learn. It not only helps you develop into a strong, confident person, but it can save you a lot of trouble in your life.

Teens start using drugs for various reasons. Whether it is because you feel unsure of yourself and look to drugs for confidence, or you're curious and want to rebel, taking a drug is not the answer to any problem.

Loss of Inhibitions

Drugs alter your personality in many ways. One common change is a loss of your inhibitions. Inhibitions are part of how you think and they control some of your activities and expressions. It may feel good to lose your inhibitions, because you think you feel more relaxed and confident without them. But you may end up doing things that you wouldn't normally do. Inhibitions can be good. They can act as warning signs to help us decide what we feel comfortable and safe doing.

When we lose our inhibitions, we may not fully weigh the consequences, or possible outcomes, of our actions. If Rachel and Eric hadn't been drinking and taking depressants, they might have decided not to have sex, or they might have been more careful and protected themselves against sexually transmitted diseases and unwanted pregnancy.

Peer Approval

Everyone wants to be liked and accepted. Most teens first try drugs when they are

20 with friends. Robert wanted people to like him, but he didn't want to take drugs. Wanting approval from his peers made it difficult for Robert to stand his ground.

Many teens start with alcohol because it is easy to find. More teenagers use alcohol than any other drug. A 1996 survey by Mothers Against Drunk Driving (MADD) estimated that about 10 million drinkers are under age twenty-one.

Taking a drink or using a drug to feel accepted and more comfortable with your friends is an easy choice to make. But in the long run, it is harmful and counter-productive. You are more likely to find success in your social life if you are yourself. If you change your personality to suit your friends or take drugs that alter your personality, you aren't being true to who you really are. It takes courage to be yourself, but it is worth it in the end.

Rebellion

It's natural to be curious about drugs. When something is forbidden, most teens want to try it even more, especially if parents are the ones saying "Don't do that. It's bad for you." It's normal to want to experience new and different things. It's

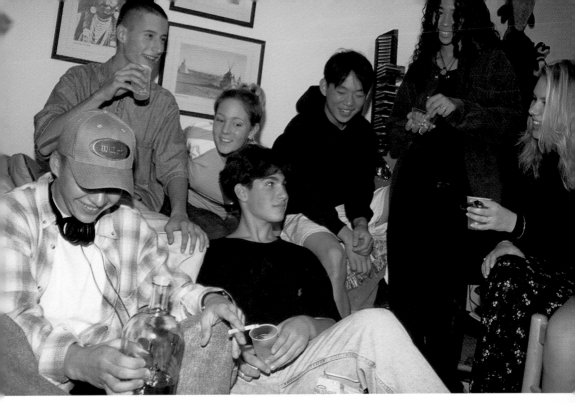

Experimenting with drugs can lead to tolerance and addiction.

also very tempting when those things pro-
mise to make you feel good.

Rebellion and experimentation are rites
of passage for most teens. But trying
drugs just to see what it feels like can be
very dangerous and lead to serious problems in your life. You can become addicted or violent, and might turn to a life
of crime to support your drug habit.
Depressant abuse is the cause of more
than half of all family violence.

Other Problems
Teens abusing drugs often don't care
about anything else. Drugs cause them to
become indifferent to their own lives as

22 well as the lives of their family and friends. Addicted teens often steal money to support their drug habit. But stealing and abusing drugs is against the law.

If you are caught taking drugs or stealing money to buy them, you are risking your future.

Due to the rise in crime by young people, many courts are giving harsher punishments to juveniles. Even if you are under eighteen years old, you may be facing jail time for drug abuse. Having a criminal record can hurt your chances of being admitted to college or getting a job.

It's important to understand what can happen to you if you use drugs—before you start using them. At the end of this book you'll find suggestions and ideas for living a drug-free life.

CHAPTER 3

Types of Depressants

*D*epressants are among the most widely used drugs in the United States. They are also the most abused. They are prescribed to treat people who suffer from anxiety, insomnia (sleeplessness), and stress. Many people are helped by depressants when they are used correctly. Prescribed by a doctor and used as directed, they can be safe.

A depressant slows down the central nervous system of the body. Depressants include barbiturates, benzodiazepines, and alcohol. Barbiturates and benzodiazepines are legal to use only with a prescription from a doctor. Alcohol is legal to use for people who are over twenty-one years of age.

23

24 | *Barbiturates*

Barbiturates are one of the two major types of depressant drugs. Barbiturates are not natural drugs; they are made in laboratories. The term "barbiturate" refers to all drugs that are made from barbituric acid. In 1862, Adolf von Baeyer created the first barbiturate by combining animal urine and acid from apples. Barbiturates were very popular in the early 1900s. Since then, more than 2,000 different types of barbiturates have been created, but only a dozen types are commonly used today.

Barbiturates usually come in powder form or as pills or capsules. They are known on the street as "downers" or "barbs." Many brands get their street names because of their colors. Nembutal pills are known as "yellow jackets." Seconal pills are called "red birds" or "red devils," and Tuinal pills are known as "rainbows" or "reds and blues."

Until the 1960s barbiturates were used safely by many people to treat anxiety disorders. An anxiety disorder causes someone to feel restless and tense. Often this anxiety causes sleeplessness. But doctors became concerned about a number of their patients who were

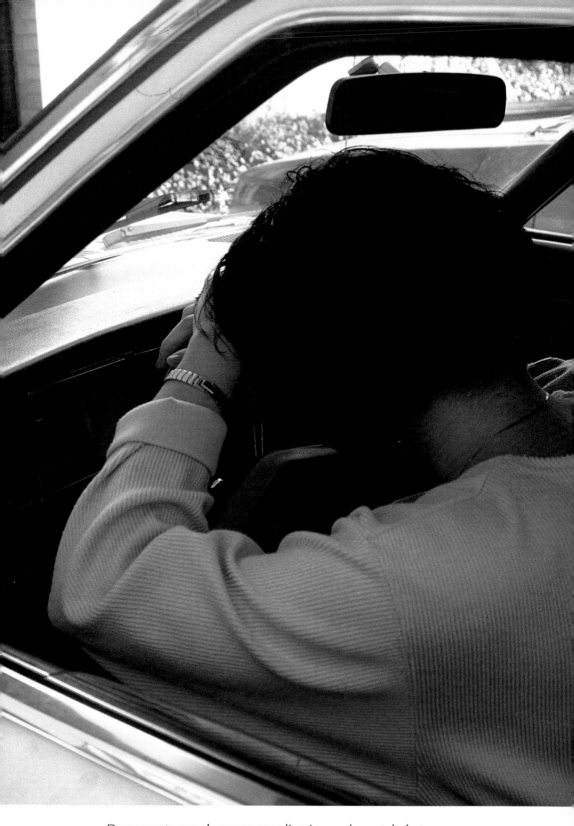

Depressants can decrease coordination and mental alertness.

26 becoming addicted to barbiturates. Some people were becoming addicted after having a legal prescription for the drug. They started out by using the depressant in a responsible way, but then became addicted to it. Others became addicted from illegal abuse of barbiturates. Overdose resulted in many deaths and led doctors to research a safer type of medication.

Today, barbiturates are mostly used for medical reasons other than anxiety disorders and insomnia. They act as an anesthetic (painkiller) in surgical procedures. They can also prevent epileptic seizures.

Benzodiazepines

Benzodiazepines were created to replace barbiturates as a treatment for anxiety and insomnia. They were developed in the 1960s and thought to be a safer alternative to barbiturates because there is less risk of death by overdose. Benzodiazepines are now commonly prescribed to treat sleeplessness and anxiety disorders. While benzodiazepines are generally safe if prescribed by a doctor and used correctly, many people abuse these drugs as well.

The most common types of benzodiazepines are Valium, Librium, and Xanax.

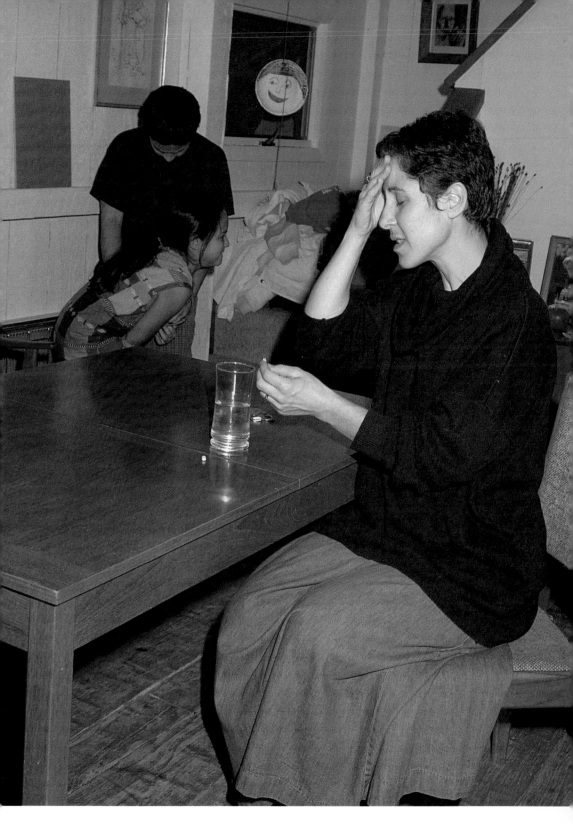

People mistakenly turn to drugs when trying to cope with the stress of daily life.

28 They are the most widely prescribed depressants in the United States. While benzodiazepines are proven to be safer than barbiturates, addiction can result in death, too. They are especially dangerous if combined with other drugs, such as narcotics like heroin and cocaine. About 50 percent of people who are treated for cocaine or heroin abuse report abusing benzodiazepines as well.

As with barbiturates, people can become addicted to benzodiazepines from prolonged medical use or illegal abuse. According to the Drug Abuse Warning Network, a 1993 analysis of hospital emergency rooms reported that 69 percent of prescription drugs misused by patients were benzodiazepines.

Abusing Barbiturates and Benzodiazepines

Abuse of barbiturates and benzodiazepines can occur in several ways. Sometimes a person uses a prescription for too long or in too high a dosage. Many people start out using a depressant in a safe and legal way, but later, after misusing the drug, lie to the doctor or persuade a doctor to write out false prescriptions.

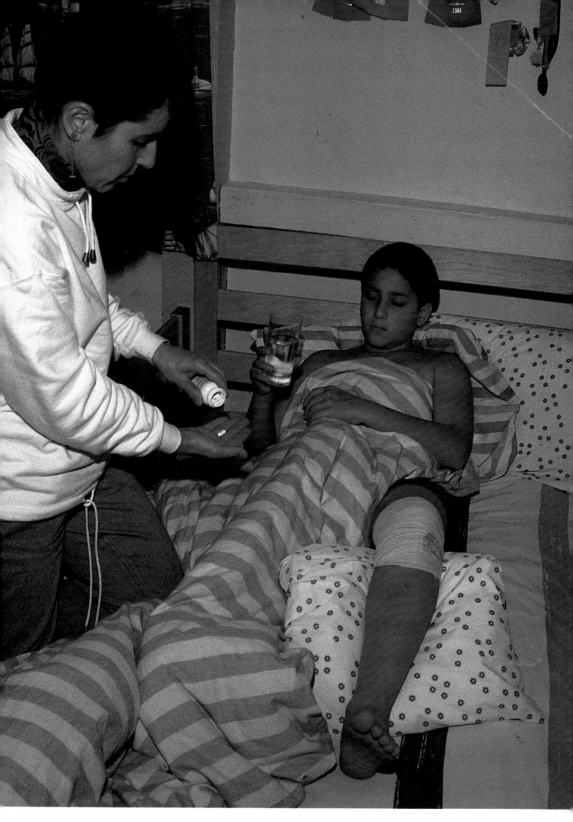

Medication that reduces pain can be safe and effective when taken as directed.

30 Then there are people who use depressants illegally just to get high. When someone takes barbiturates or benzodiazepines illegally without a prescription, he or she may start out with small amounts. But soon the amount needed to get high increases, and addiction is likely to follow. Some drug dealers steal doctors' prescription pads so they can get prescriptions filled. Some dealers even steal drugs from pharmacies. These illegally obtained drugs wind up being sold on the street.

Even though the process of addiction may be different for the prescribed user and the illegal user, the dangers of addiction are the same. Addiction to depressants is more dangerous than addiction to any other kind of drug. The withdrawal symptoms of these drugs are life threatening. Stopping without medical help can cause seizures and other medical problems that can result in coma or death. If you or someone you know is addicted, be sure to get medical help. A doctor's supervision is needed to quit both barbiturates and benzodiazepines.

Alcohol

Alcohol is also a depressant. It has been around for centuries. Before modern medicine, it was used to ease tension and help put people to sleep. At one time, it was also the only drug doctors could give to a patient to ease the pain of surgery. Today, it is no longer used for medicinal purposes.

Alcohol is used and enjoyed in a responsible way by many people, but many others abuse it. Some people drink alcohol for the same reasons that others take barbiturates and benzodiazepines. Alcohol makes them feel relaxed and happy.

A responsible drinker knows what alcohol does to the body and drinks with caution. Drinking alcohol with caution means more than knowing how much you should or shouldn't drink. It also means knowing when and where it's okay to drink. Because alcohol is legal, teens may think that it is always safe. But alcohol can be very dangerous if abused. That's why the law says you must be over twenty-one years of age to drink. Alcohol causes over 500 deaths every day in the United States.

As with other depressants, it is easy to develop a tolerance for alcohol and begin abusing it. Abusing alcohol can mean drinking too much or needing to drink to face difficult situations. Abusing alcohol

32 | can progress into the disease of alco-
holism. An alcoholic is a person who
cannot control his or her drinking. When
an alcoholic starts drinking, he or she
cannot stop. More people are addicted to
alcohol than any other depressant.

Alcoholism

Some of the warning signs of alcoholism
include:

- preoccupation with alcohol—taking
  part only in activities that include
  alcohol;
- need for a drink to relax or get to
  sleep;
- increase of tolerance to the point of
  not appearing drunk even after
  drinking a lot of alcohol;
- loss of control over drinking—
  inability to stop after one drink;
- solitary drinking;
- blackouts—not remembering what
  happened after drinking.

An alcoholic who suddenly stops
drinking also suffers severe withdrawal
symptoms. It's important to consult
with a doctor to see if medical help is
necessary to quit. The severe symptoms

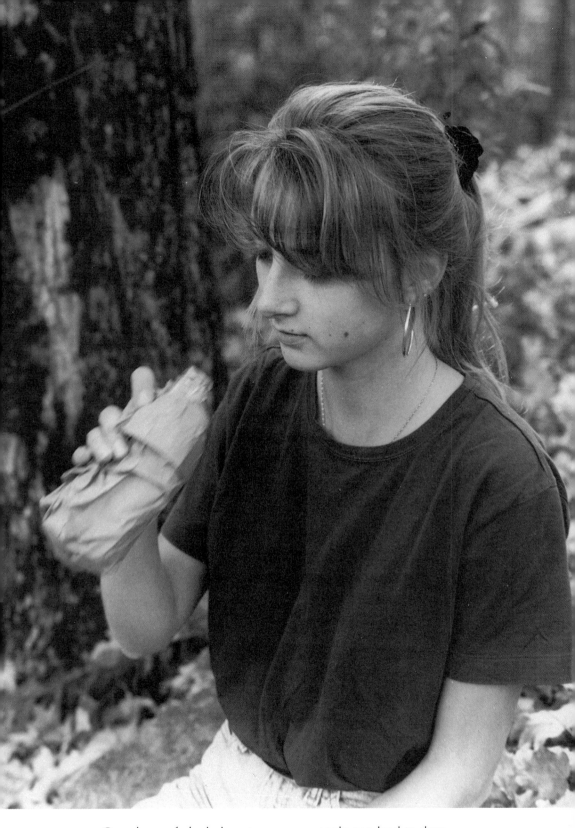

Casual use of alcohol among young people can lead to drug abuse and addiction.

34 generally last only a few days, although discomfort can last for many weeks.

While it is possible to use depressant drugs in a safe, responsible way, you need to be aware of the effects of abuse and addiction. Addiction to barbiturates, benzodiazepines, and alcohol is extremely dangerous. If you are addicted and you try to stop without medical help, you may die.

CHAPTER 4

The Effects of Depressants

*B*rian was in love with Lee Ann. He had known her since childhood and hoped to marry her one day. But over the last year, their relationship had become very unsteady. Lee Ann had started taking Valium because she had trouble sleeping.

When her prescription expired after a few weeks, she changed doctors and kept getting more and more Valium. Sometimes, she would fake a prescription. She often took the Valium with beer or wine. Brian wanted very much to help her. If she couldn't make it to school, he brought her the assignments and sometimes did them for her. If she needed money, he gave it to her. He even went to the pharmacy to refill her prescriptions.

Brian wanted Lee Ann to be happy, and she got really angry if he didn't help her out when she felt sick. Brian was afraid Lee Ann would leave him if he didn't make her happy. His whole life began to revolve around Lee Ann and her problems.

Depressants affect the central nervous system and cause the body and brain to slow down. They depress normal body and brain functions. As soon as they enter the bloodstream, they lower the blood pressure, heart, and breathing activity. Because of their effects, an overdose (taking too much of the drug) can be fatal.

Physical Effects

When someone takes a depressant, he or she feels very relaxed. This feeling may cause the user to feel high, even though a depressant slows the body down. Later effects include slurred speech, loss of inhibitions, and slowed reactions. The eyes become lazy, move jerkily, and have difficulty focusing.

Depressants cause more than half of all accidental poisonings. That is because many abusers do not realize that these drugs can have a multiplying effect when taken with other depressants. For example, if someone drinks alcohol and takes a barbiturate, the effect may be ten times stronger than that of either the barbiturate or the alcohol taken alone.

Depressants produce severe withdrawal symptoms, including anxiety, insomnia, tremors, delirium, convulsions, and possible death. These withdrawal symptoms contribute to the dangerous cycle of depressant abuse. That is, abusers take more drugs to avoid suffering withdrawal symptoms. Physical dependence on barbiturates is one of the most dangerous of all drug dependencies.

Barbiturates and benzodiazepines, more than other drugs, become more dangerous with each use. Every time abusers increase the amount of any such drug, they come closer to the point at which the drug can kill them. The higher the person's tolerance, the higher the risk for overdose and death. Although the body develops a tolerance for the intoxicating effects, it does not have a tolerance for the lethal effects. Therefore, when the tolerance increases, the body craves more of the drug to feel a certain way; but that doesn't mean the body can handle larger amounts. An addict may overdose trying to achieve the earlier effect.

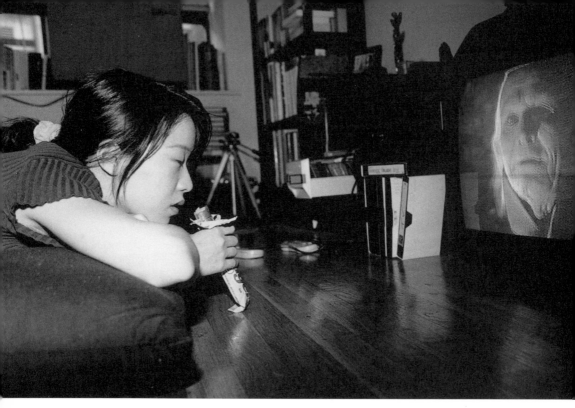

The physical effects of depressants include slurred speech, drowsiness, and slowed reactions.

Psychological Effects

Depressant abusers claim that the drugs make them feel at peace, happy, sexy, friendly, relaxed, uninhibited, confident, fearless, and without pain.

When depressants are abused over a long period of time, they affect a person's judgment and memory. They cause mood swings, depression, and fatigue. Depressants can also cause the user to feel paranoid or have suicidal thoughts.

Friends and family members are
usually the first to notice that something

is different about the depressant abuser.
The changes are severe. When abusers
become addicts, they reach a point at
which they don't care much about anything—not their families, friends, school-
work, appearance, pets, or job. Certainly,
they do not care as much about any of
these things as they do about depressants.

Denial
One of the main psychological problems
experienced by a drug abuser is denial.
Denial is the act of unconsciously ignor-
ing a problem in order to avoid dealing
with it.

Addicts are often in denial. When an
addict is in denial, he or she insists the
drug use is under control. An addict's
family may also be in denial because they
refuse to believe their loved one has a
problem. With treatment, an addict and
his or her family can come to accept the
problem and work to overcome it.

Depression
Addicts are often depressed and ashamed
of the addiction. Addicts have lost control
over their lives. They cannot stop abusing
drugs and often cannot even admit that
there is a problem. They may also be

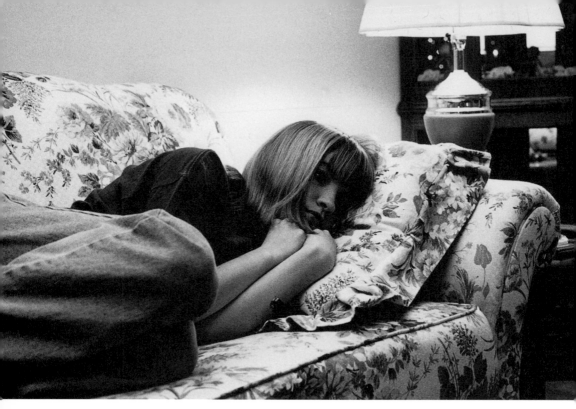

Addicts often suffer from depression and severe mood swings.

afraid to stop because the withdrawal symptoms are so severe. This fear causes addicts to continue taking the drugs. They are caught in a terrible cycle of abuse, depression, and more abuse.

Codependency

As a person's drug abuse gets worse, the lives of his or her family and friends are negatively affected. It's difficult to watch someone you love and care about be hurt by drugs. A friend or family member may become an enabler. An enabler is someone who unknowingly supports the addict's habit. Enablers try to help by controlling the addict's behavior.

For example, a wife may call in sick for her hungover husband because she's afraid he'll lose his job. A boyfriend may do his girlfriend's homework when she misses school, so she won't fail the class. A mother may give her child money, even though she knows the child uses it to buy drugs. This kind of codependent behavior by family members and friends prevents the addict from seeing how destructive his or her behavior really is.

An enabler becomes obsessed with trying to get the addict to stop abusing drugs. But by trying to control the addict's behavior, he or she allows the abuse to continue. Only an addict can admit to having the disease. Only an addict can make the decision to stop using. And only after facing the negative consequences of drug use will he or she realize the problem. The longer an enabler is involved, the longer it takes for the addict to reach this realization.

CHAPTER 5

Getting Help

*I*f you or someone you know has been abusing depressants, it's very important to get help. The first step to getting help is talking to someone who can support you. It's important to talk to someone you can trust. Here are some of the people you can turn to.

Your Parents
Parents care about their children. They may be upset because of your drug abuse, but they want to help you. Most parents can be counted on to do their best for you. If you are ready to stop using, your parents will probably give you the support you need and make sure you get medical

help. You might start by giving them this book to read.

If your parents can't or won't help, don't give up. Other people can give you the help you need.

Your Teacher

Talk to a teacher you trust. If your teacher doesn't know exactly what to do, he or she usually does know how to find out. He or she can put you in touch with a professional who can help you. If you don't have a teacher you feel comfortable talking with, go to the next person on your list.

Your School Counselor

Counselors are specially trained to help young people like you. It's their job. Many of them know a lot about depressants. Some of them will be acquainted with the kinds of services available in your community.

Religious Leader

Religious leaders can be great sources of help. Some are familiar with the problems of addiction and will be eager to help. Others may know exactly where to refer you for help. They can also give you ideas

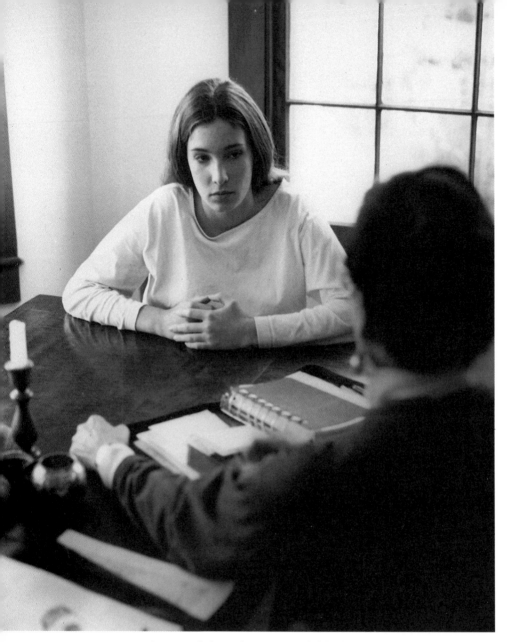

Help to end drug abuse is available from a variety of agencies and counselors.

on how to tell your parents. They may even be willing to go with you when you tell your parents.

A word of warning is needed, however. If your religious leader tells you that

prayer alone will get rid of your

addiction, find someone else to consult. Remember, you need medical help in order to get off depressants.

Crisis and Drug Hot Lines

In larger cities, telephone counseling services have been established for the purpose of helping youth. They are usually staffed by people who understand alcohol and drug abuse. They should know where the best services are for someone in your situation. They may even be able to make an appointment and arrange transportation for you to see a doctor.

Some of these phone services are staffed by peer counselors. These are people your own age who have been trained to help others. You may find it easier to discuss your problem with a peer. In any case, be sure to tell the person with whom you speak everything you can about the types and amounts of depressants you have been using, and any problems you are having.

Certified Alcohol and Drug Counselor (CADC)

CADCs are professionals in the drug and alcohol field. They spend their lives helping people who are addicted. They can

46 help you in more ways than anyone else.

CADCs are trained to counsel persons who are addicted to drugs and alcohol. They can help you talk to your parents about the problem. They can also help you decide what steps to take to overcome your addiction.

To find a CADC, look in the Yellow Pages of the telephone directory under Alcoholism or Drug Counselors. You will find the letters CADC written after the counselors' names.

If you have been using depressants and have stopped for a day or two, your body could be going into withdrawal. The symptoms of withdrawal are nausea, extreme nervousness, shakiness, stomach cramps, excessive sweating, convulsions, or delirium (seeing, hearing, or feeling things that are not there). If you experience any of these symptoms, call 9-1-1 immediately.

CHAPTER 6

Choosing to Quit

*L*ee Ann eventually hit rock bottom when Brian broke up with her. He said that he could no longer watch her destroy her life and stopped filling her prescriptions. Lee Ann was making her family miserable with worry. She left home and stopped going to school altogether. When she couldn't find a place to stay, Lee Ann was a wreck. She didn't know what to do.

Lee Ann saw a drug hot line advertised on television and decided to call. She talked to a trained counselor. The counselor told her to check herself into the hospital. Lee Ann was scared. She was already suffering from some withdrawal symptoms. The counselor *urged Lee Ann to call her parents and ask them to take her to the hospital for treatment. It was difficult to do, but her parents were relieved when she called. They told her they would support her as best they could. Lee Ann had made the first step toward recovery.*

It's not easy to quit abusing any drug. Depressants can be even more difficult because you need medical supervision to stop. The withdrawal symptoms of barbiturates and benzodiazepines are very dangerous. Addicts should not try to quit these drugs without medical help. If an addict tries to stop alone, his or her life is at risk.

While quitting depressants is not easy, making the choice to quit will save your life.

Because many people who are addicted to drugs can't afford treatment, special programs are available to help low-income patients. If you or someone you know needs help, contact your local public health department. They will tell you whom to contact for help in your area. There are hot lines listed at the end of this book that will also tell you what services are available to you.

Once a person is addicted to depressants, he or she may be afraid to try to quit. Going into the hospital can sound scary. It's important to remember, though, that quitting is worth it. Drug addiction destroys any normal life you can have. Quitting will give you your life back.

It's also important to know what happens when you decide to quit. Understanding the process will help you overcome your fear. The process of overcoming physical dependency is the first step.

Withdrawal

When an addict stops using drugs, he or she experiences withdrawal symptoms. Depending on the drug, withdrawal can begin at different times after the last use. For example, withdrawal from alcohol can occur from twelve to forty-eight hours after the last drink. Barbiturate withdrawal usually occurs seventy-two hours after the last dose. Benzodiazepines may take a week or more to produce withdrawal symptoms. The effects of withdrawal are the worst after a long period of abuse. There are three main stages of depressant withdrawal.

50   The first stage of withdrawal can include sleeping problems, anxiety, low fever, and agitation.

The second stage includes all the symptoms of the first plus hallucinations. Hallucinations are seeing and hearing things that aren't really there. The second stage can also include vomiting and body tremors.

The third stage is the most dangerous. It includes a high fever and severe disorientation. With disorientation, a person fails to recognize known objects or people. There is general confusion about time and place as well. At this stage, an addict needs emergency medical help. This is also the stage when most deaths occur.

When you decide to stop using, you need to check yourself into a hospital immediately. Do it before the symptoms of withdrawal start.

Hospital Treatment

After entering the hospital, a patient is evaluated physically and mentally. The patient is tested to determine exactly what drugs are being abused. Unfortunately, addicts often lie about the extent of their drug use. Addicts lie to defend

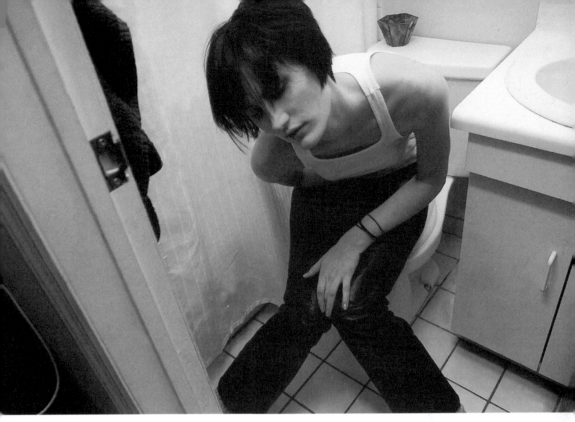

Withdrawal symptoms can make a user feel sick.

the continuing use of the drugs. This behavior is also called minimizing. Addicts minimize their drug use because it's too painful to accept the truth. It's necessary to determine what drugs are in a patient's system before withdrawal treatment can begin.

Treating physical dependence involves a process called detoxification. Detoxification means freeing the body of the addictive substance. The treatment is designed to prevent withdrawal stages two and

52 | three. Treatment also tries to prevent the patient from having seizures. The process can be handled in two different ways.

In the first way, a doctor reduces the amount of the drug the patient is taking. Under careful supervision, the patient is given smaller and smaller doses of the drug. It is a step-by-step process. The goal is to lessen the effects of the withdrawal symptoms while completely freeing the body of the drug.

In the second way, a doctor may choose to give the patient a substitute drug. The substitute drug has the same effects as the depressant, but has a lower risk of severe withdrawal symptoms. This substitute drug is also given in gradually smaller doses until the patient is no longer physically dependent on it. Careful guidance is also needed, however, to be sure the patient does not become dependent on the substitute drug. For example, an alcoholic may be given a benzodiazepine during detoxification. The benzodiazepine helps the addict through the withdrawal process, but it is very important to ensure that the patient doesn't become dependent on the benzodiazepine.

Staying off Drugs   53

Once the body has safely gone through the detoxification process, it is time to address the psychological aspects of addiction. In order for a patient to successfully stay off drugs, it is essential that he or she make some major life changes.

It is necessary for a patient to undergo therapy to talk about what has happened. Recovering addicts need to understand the results of their behavior in order to learn how to avoid any obstacles to recovery. One of the changes recovering addicts need to make is to stay away from the places and people involved in their drug abuse. They need to find drug-free, supportive friends, along with new, drug-free activities.

The beginning of recovery is a very difficult and frightening time. It is hard to confront the past and face the future. The past is filled with bad behavior and the hopelessness that comes with drug addiction. The future is a long process of recovery that, at times, may seem impossible. Sometimes addicts relapse. Relapse means a person starts using drugs again shortly after detoxification. When someone suffers a relapse, it is usually

54 | because he or she does not have the proper support system.

Recovery Programs

If you are committed to quitting, and have taken the first steps to recovery, you can stay off drugs. It's important to remember, however, that hospitalization alone is not enough. An addict also needs a recovery program. Groups such as Alcoholics Anonymous and Narcotics Anonymous offer help. Their programs give patients tools for recovery. Participants learn new types of behavior and receive support from others who have had similar experiences.

CHAPTER 7

Living a Drug-Free Lifestyle

*R*obert doesn't hang around with Jeremy anymore. He got tired of going to parties and watching Jeremy and his friends drink and do drugs. He didn't want to start using drugs and end up like Jeremy, but he also didn't want people to think he was uncool.

In early spring, Robert joined the track team. The coach thought he had potential and encouraged him to think about trying to get a running scholarship to help him afford college. Robert started hanging out with some of the students on the team. He found that taking good care of his body helped him run faster and longer. Robert began to feel really good about himself and his accomplishments.

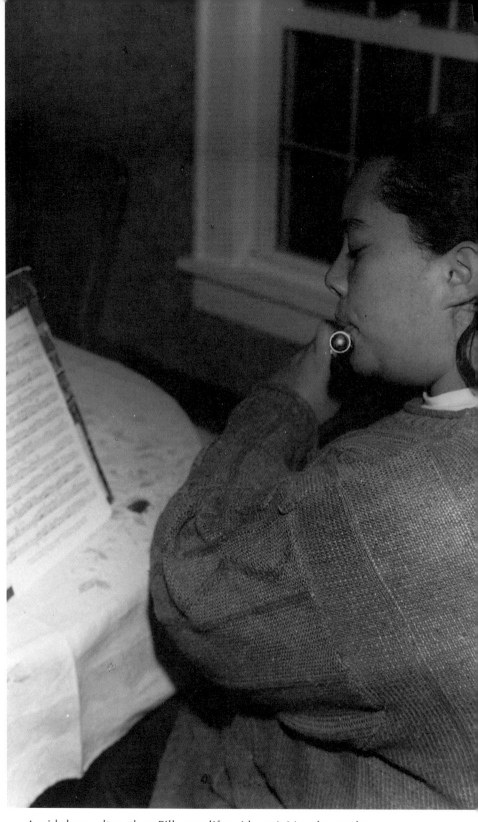

Avoid drugs altogether. Fill your life with activities that make
you feel good about yourself.

The best choice you can make for yourself is not to use drugs. That's not an easy choice in today's fast-moving world, but it's one worth making. Drugs steal away any control you have over your life. Before you try any drug, think about all that you have to lose. Take responsibility for your life and do something positive that makes you feel good about yourself. Robert found that running gave him a natural high and increased his self-esteem. He made an investment in himself and his future by choosing not to do drugs.

Drugs and the temptation to experiment with them will always be around. But making the choice not to do them will become easier and easier each time you say no. This choice will save you from a lot of pain and misery, and it will give you a more fulfilling life.

Glossary—
Explaining New Words

addiction   Inability to stop using alcohol or other mind-altering drugs.

central nervous system   The brain and spinal cord, which direct all of the body's activities.

denial   Psychological defense mechanism of refusing to admit a problem.

dependence   The state of relying on an addictive substance.

detoxification   Medical process of freeing the body of all traces of drugs.

disorientation   Loss of the sense of time and place; mental confusion.

enabler   Person who makes it possible for an addict or abuser to maintain the disability by making excuses for him or her.

inhibition An inner barrier to certain kinds of expression or activity.

peers Persons of same social group by either age or status.

rite of passage An activity associated with a change of status (such as from adolescence to adulthood).

tolerance The body's developing ability to adjust to increasing quantities of an addictive substance.

withdrawal Stopping the use of an addictive drug and the physical symptoms that go along with stopping.

Where to Go for Help

**Al-Anon/Alateen Family Group
 Headquarters, Inc.**
P.O. Box 862, Midtown Station
New York, NY 10018
(800) 443-4525

American Council for Drug Education
204 Monroe Street
Rockville, MD 20852
(301) 294-0600

Benzodiazepine Anonymous
6333 Wilshire Boulevard, Suite 506
Los Angeles, CA 90048
(310) 652-4100

Nar-Anon Family Groups
P.O. Box 2562
Palos Verdes Peninsula, CA 91406
(310) 547-5800

National Association of Children of Alcoholics

11426 Rockville Pike, Suite 100
Rockville, MD 20852
(301) 468-0985
Web site: http://ww.health.org.nacoa

National Clearinghouse for Alcohol and Drug Information

P.O. Box 2345
Rockville, MD 20852
(301) 468-2600

National Council on Alcoholism and Drug Dependency (NCADD)

12 West 21st Street
New York, NY 10010
(800) 662-HELP
Web site: http://www.ncadd.org/

For Further Reading

Ball, J. *Everything You Need to Know About Drug Abuse.* New York: The Rosen Publishing Group, 1990.

Berger, G. *The Pressure to Take Drugs.* New York: Franklin Watts, 1990.

Clayton, L. *Working Together Against Drug Addiction.* New York: The Rosen Publishing Group, 1996.

Edwards, G. *Coping with Drug Abuse.* New York: The Rosen Publishing Group, 1990.

Leite, E., and P. Espeland. *Different Like Me.* Minneapolis: Johnson Institute, 1987.

McFarland, R. *Coping with Substance Abuse.* New York: The Rosen Publishing Group, 1990.

Porterfield, K. *Coping with an Alcoholic Parent.* New York: The Rosen Publishing Group, 1991.

Index

About the Author

Dr. Lawrence Clayton earned his doctorate from Texas Woman's University. He is an ordained minister and has served as such since 1972. Dr. Clayton is a clinical marriage and family therapist and certified drug and alcohol counselor. He is also president of the Oklahoma Professional Drug and Alcohol Counselor's Certification Board. Dr. Clayton lives with his wife, Cathy, and their three children in Piedmont, Oklahoma.

Photo Credits

Cover Photo: Stuart Rabinowitz
Photo on page 8: Katherine Hsu; photo on page 21: Ira Fox; photo on page 38: Michael Brandt; photo on page 40: John Novajosky; photo on page 51: Sarah Friedman. All other photos by Stuart Rabinowitz.